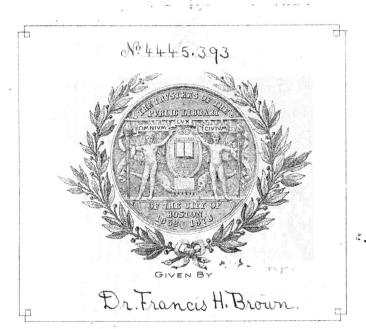

DR. SAMUEL FULLER, OF THE MAYFLOWER (1620), THE PIONEER PHYSICIAN.

By THOMAS F. HARRINGTON, M. D., of *Lowell, Mass.*

[From The Johns Hopkins Hospital Bulletin, Vol. XIV, No. 151,
October, 1903.]

DR. SAMUEL FULLER, OF THE MAYFLOWER (1620), THE PIONEER PHYSICIAN.*

By Thomas F. Harrington, M. D., *of Lowell, Mass.*

There is no epoch in modern history more eventful to the [263] medical profession than that marking the closing of the sixteenth and the beginning of the seventeenth centuries. The discovery of America, the extension of the printing-press, the awakening of scientific thought and inquiry, all foretold a new era in the world's history, which should forever stand forth illumining by its warm rays all future ages. The light of reason and skepticism was to be as destructive to the demon theory of disease which had prevailed from the Middle Ages as its stimulating influences were to be beneficial to progress and advancement. The age found the man, and from the University of Basel (1526) the clear voice of Paracelsus (1493-1541) rings forth bidding the fettered mind to awake and come out of the darkness. Truly this was a wonderful man. However much we may find to condemn in his teachings and methods, his truths will ever serve as the foundation to successful medicine. "Reading never made a doctor," he said, "but practice is what forms a physician. For all reading is a foot-stool to practice, and a mere feather broom. He who meditates discovers something." Again he says, "The book of nature was that which the physician should read, and to do so he must walk over its leaves." His ætiology of diseases was divided into five causes: foul air, errors in digestion and assimilation, diathesis, disorders due to perverted ideas, and lastly diseases due to causes predetermined by God.[1]

---

* Read before the Johns Hopkins Historical Club, April 20, 1903.

(1)

[263] His discoveries included metal zinc and hydrogen gas; he invented laudanum; and he anticipated the transfusion of blood; he substituted tinctures and quintessence of drugs for the filthy masses and unscientific mixtures; he introduced mercury for the treatment of syphilis, and the use of iron, sulphur, antimony, arsenic, tin and lead, as well as baths, also arnica and other vegetable remedies in the treatment of disease; he revolutionized the barbarous treatment of dislocations and fractures, honor enough, one might think, for one man. Greatly as it would profit us to dwell at some length upon the life and works of Paracelsus, the purpose of introducing him here is to point out the influence at work in the scientific world tending to produce abundant good fruit. For this result we do not look in vain. Electricity, chemistry, mineralogy, botany and pharmacy all advanced rapidly, each giving its due quota to medicine for the betterment and uplifting of mankind.' The medical profession received its first legislative recognition by Parliament (1511), physicians and surgeons were exempted by law (1542) from military and jury duty in order that they might be the freer to attend to their duties, colleges for the instruction of medical students were established, and laws against irregular practitioners and quacks were enacted (1542).' The labors and investigations of Vesalius (1514-1564), Fallopius (1523-1562), [264] Eustachius (1510-1574), Servetus (1511-1553), and Ambroise Parè (1517-1590) had awakened the medical mind to the study of anatomy, physiology and surgery such as had never been done before, and plainly foretold almost to anticipation the great discovery of Harvey (1578-1657) which meant the establishment of the theory and practice of medicine upon a new and permanent foundation. Kepler (1571-1630), Galileo (1564-1642), Reubens (1577-1640), Francis Bacon (1561-1626), and Shakspear (1564-1616) were entering upon the world's stage, there to leave, each in his own sphere, a model which would stand for all ages. Providence seems to have decreed that from that age one should be born whom the followers in the new world of His works as exemplified by the Apostle Luke should find worthy of emulating.

Samuel Fuller was baptized at Redenhall Parish

Church, in Norfolk county, England, January 20, 1580.' [264]
He was the son of Robert Fuller, who is registered as
a butcher, which was ranked with the trades and professions.
That the Fullers were prominent people in the parish for more
than one hundred years prior to Samuel Fuller's birth is evident from the records. Unfortunately the custom of that age
did not include mentioning the name of the mother in the
registry of births, consequently little is known of Mrs. Fuller's
ancestry. Information as to the early life and doings of young
Fuller is very meagre. It is stated, however, that he had been
a silk worker,' whether as an apprentice to some Frenchman
as his friend and companion William Bradford was, can only
be conjectured; positive it is, however, that at some time in
early youth these two young men formed a companionship
which makes it impossible to consider their lives separately.
Samuel Fuller's marked career began at Leyden, where he
is early spoken of as one of the deacons of that church'
which was soon to play such an important part in the settlement of the new world. This office of deacon was not
an empty one, for the deacons of the church, though lay-
men, were as carefully selected and formally ordained as
the clergymen. Previous to coming to Leyden he had married
Elsie Glascock, probably in England,' who lived but a short
time, and in 1613, according to Leyden records, he married
Agnes, daughter of Alexander Carpenter, a family of such
superior position that the suit of William Bradford for the
hand in marriage of another daughter, Alice, was not looked
upon with favor, notwithstanding the fact that Bradford
belonged to the two best families in his section. Bradford
afterwards married Alice in America (August 14, 1623).
Soon death again robbed Deacon Fuller of his wife, and he
married his third and last wife, Bridget, daughter of Mrs.
Joseph Lee, at Leyden, 1617.

Of his life at Leyden much is known. He was reckoned
as one of the persons of large means,' and both on account
of his blood and marriage connections with many of the
leading families of Rev. John Robinson's congregation, as well
as the power of his own force of character, he early became an
active and important factor in the affairs of that band of

Separatists.[8] Fuller joined the Scrooby band of Pilgrims at Leyden in 1609, where they had gone after leaving Amsterdam. This settlement included William Bradford, John Robinson, William Brewster, Isaac Allerton, Edward Winslow, John Carver, Miles Standish, William White, as well as others, all of whose names to-day are so familiar in the history of the first settlements in this country. In the negotiations and preparations for fitting out the Speedwell and the Mayflower (1617-1620) Fuller was an active and influential party.[9] He was the first signer to the letter written jointly by Fuller, Winslow, Brewster and Allerton to Carver and Cushman, date June 10 (new style), 1620, in which they sharply criticise Cushman's actions in his dealings with the Virginia Company and later with "the Merchant Adventurers" while acting as the agent for the Pilgrims.

For more than twenty years prior to the emigration of the Pilgrims from Leyden the Puritanic clergy were educated to the medical profession [10] in anticipation of their pilgrimage which persecution at home was surely forcing upon them. Oxford, too, foreseeing the difficulties in store for the clergy, incorporated the study of physic in the course for the divinity student. A part of this education consisted in the study of the ancient medical authors, as Hippocrates, Galen, Breteus, Celsus and others. Thus it was that many clergymen were eminent practitioners of medicine before they crossed the Atlantic, where necessity often forced the two duties into one. William Brewster, with whom Fuller was closely associated at Leyden, was a man of great learning and ability. In his capacity as secretary to Davison, one of Elizabeth's ambassadors and secretary of state, Brewster had many opportunities for study. He became a noted teacher and so magnetic was his style that students from all quarters came to the famous Leyden University to partake of his knowledge. His methods attracted the attention of many of the eminent men of that period. Bradford speaks of Leyden as "a fair & bewtifull citie, and of a sweet situation, but made more famous by ye universitie wherwith it is adorned, in which of late had been so many learned men." Fuller was indeed fortunate in having the friendship and association of this

man, especially at Leyden, and at a time when great discover- [264]
ies were being made in the field of medicine. In 1616 Harvey
first expounded to his students the circulation of the blood
which he published to the world twelve years later. [11] Aided
by the discovery of the microscope in 1621, the doctrine of
Harvey on the development of the higher animals from the
ovum, as well as the acceptance of his description of the circulation of the blood, a new era was commenced in medical
science which meant a complete overthrow of the followers
of the Ancients, and one which effected a total revolution
in the theory and practice of medicine. The science of medicine became greatly interwoven with the science of philosophy,
thus broadening the human mind. Investigation and experi-
ment supplanted dogmatism and blind faith; human dissec-
tion which had slept for fifteen centuries was revived; anatomy and physiology were studied by means of actual dissections; many new remedies were introduced in the treatment
of disease, including lemon juice for scurvy, Peruvian bark
for malaria, as well as sarsaparilla and guaiacum. The instruction of medical students in England was mostly confined [265]
to the guilds, and consisted of lectures and demonstrations in
dissections for which the government furnished bodies. Be-
sides these compulsory lectures there were many private and
endowed courses. Harvey was lecturer for forty-one years
(1616-1656) in one of these courses (the Lumleian [12]), and it
was here that he first made known his discovery. Medical
publications were scarce and subjected to the closest censor-
ship. Surgeons and barbers were now recognized as separate
bodies.

Surrounded by such conditions and afforded every oppor-
tunity to take the fullest advantages of his privileges, it is
but reasonable to suppose that an active, energetic, studious
mind, such as we know Samuel Fuller to have possessed, must
of necessity become well equipped for his chosen work. In
forming an estimate of Doctor Fuller two sources of error
confront us. First we are apt to consider him as a clergyman who had studied medicine and who was not a regularly
educated physician, and secondly the too commonly accepted
belief that superstition, astrology and ignorance predomi-

nated at that time. Now as to the first it can be positively said that while he was well educated in clerical matters, his profession was medicine, and it was as physician and not as minister that he came to America. There is perhaps no stronger proof of this than the words of Pastor Robinson in his final letter to his brother-in-law, John Carver, just before the Mayflower sailed (July 27, 1620). He says:[13] ". . . I have written a large letter to ye whole, and am sorrie I shall not rather speak than write to them, & the more considering ye want of a preacher, which I shall also make sume spurr to my hastening after you. . . ." In the list of the passengers sailing on the Mayflower the occupation of Samuel Fuller is given as Physician, and "the vocations given were, as far as ascertained, the callings the individuals who represented them had followed before taking ship."[14] Dr. Thacher in his memoirs says:[15] "The first physician of whom we have any account among the Colonists was Dr. Samuel Fuller. . . . Whether he had enjoyed a collegiate education is uncertain, but he is said to have been well qualified in his profession; he was zealous in the cause of religion, and eminently useful as a physician and surgeon." An account of the sickness in Governor Endicott's Settlement at Salem in 1628 says:[16] "Having no physician among themselves, it was fortunate for those planters that Plymouth could supply them with one so well qualified as Dr. Fuller." From these accounts as well as the numerous evidences of his learning and skill found in his life and labors in this country, it must be acknowledged that Dr. Samuel Fuller was a worthy representative of the medical profession of that period.

Previous to the coming of the Mayflower, Dr. Wotton (1606), Dr. Russell (1607) and Dr. Bagnall (1608) had accompanied expeditions to Virginia, and served as surgeon to Captain John Smith's party. History does not record how long they remained in this country. That none of them settled here would seem positive from the account given by Smith, who says[17] that he was compelled to return to Europe for the recovery of his health in 1609 after being badly wounded by the explosion of gunpowder, as there was neither chirurgeon nor chirurgery at the fort. In 1610 Dr. Bohun

came to this country, and in 1611 he accompanied Lord Dela-
ware to the West Indies. He was killed in a fight with a
Spanish warship. It has been said that the Mayflower had a
surgeon (Giles Heale), but nothing is recorded about him
other than his signature to William Mullins' will. Mullins
died February, 1621, on the Mayflower. There is no other
mention of this surgeon either as a passenger or sailor on
board the Mayflower. Therefore I think that it can be positively said that Dr. Samuel Fuller was the first physician to
settle in the colonies and the pioneer English-speaking physician of this country.

As to the mental outfit of the early colonists much might
be said, praiseworthy and otherwise. Astrology was the science that touched the popular imagination. Medicines were
given when the moon was in the proper sign; horoscopic
diagnoses were common practices; weaning of infants on the
proper sign of the zodiac was the rule, all remnants of the
influences surviving from the Middle Ages. Superstition had
its believers even among the educated, yet the very influences
thought to be the greatest hindrance to advancement, namely,
the lack of opportunities for book learning, the absence of
newspapers, periodicals and journals to spread the knowledge
gained as well as the exigent wants of the people, were all
factors in compelling close observation in their new surround-
ings, and a keen stimulant to the desire for schools and
churches upon which to build a government indestructible.
That Doctor Fuller was one of those equipped with the mental training suitable to enable him to make the best of his
new environment must be admitted. In a time when the
very suspicion of possessing medical skill made it dangerous
to be thus recognized it speaks strongly of Dr. Fuller's courage
and high-mindedness to be looked upon as the one person
best qualified in the knowledge of medicine. A small ship
of about 60 tons was fitted out in Holland and was to accom-
pany the Mayflower to this country. Dr. Fuller was evi-
dently not a passenger on this ill-fated ship, for an account
of the sailing (about July 22, 1620) says:[18] "just who of the
Leyden chiefs caused themselves to be assigned to the small
vessel (Speedwell) to encourage its cowardly Weston cannot

[265] be definitely known. It may be confidently assumed, however, that Dr. Samuel Fuller the physician of the colonists was transferred to the Mayflower upon which were embarked 3/4ths of the entire company, including most of the women and children, with some of whom it was evident his services would be certainly in demand." There appears to have been very little sickness, other than seasickness, among the passengers during that long and trying voyage. One of the seamen, an able-bodied man much given to profanity, was stricken with a "grieveous disease of which he dyed in a desperate manner, and was ye first yt was throwne overboard." [19] Whether this was a case of delirium tremens [20] no positive knowledge exists. Two weeks later on the day before land was sighted the second death occurred. This was William
[266] Butten, the servant-student to Dr. Fuller, and he was the only passenger who died on the voyage. Dr. Fuller, unlike all the other leaders, did not bring his wife and family with him. His only attendant was the youth Butten who is designated in the Log Book as "servant-assistant to Dr. Fuller." The fact that there was very little sickness on the Mayflower speaks well for the physical condition of the party, which is said by Winslow "to be the youngest and strongest of the Leyden congregation." That there were troubles other than sicknesses against which the leaders had to contend would appear from the following: "This day before we came to harbor observing some not well affected to unity and concord, but gave some appearance of faction, it was thought good there should be an association and agreement that we should combine together in one body, and to submit to such government and Governors as we should, by common consent, agree to make and choose, and set our hands to this that follows word for word." [21] This dissatisfaction arose on account of the abandonment of the location for settlement on territory under the protection of the patent granted by the London Virginia Company. Consequently on the 11th day of November, 1620, all the adult male passengers except two seamen, and those too ill, met in the cabin of the Mayflower and there drew up and signed the famous compact, a basis

of civil self-government fame of which will never die. Sam-
uel Fuller was the eighth signer of this memorable declaration. He was preceded in order by, first, John Carver; second, William Bradford, the leader and guide; third, Edward Winslow, the diplomat; fourth, William Brewster, the elder and scholar; fifth, Isaac Allerton, the active, progressive business man; sixth, Miles Standish, the Cincinnatus of the colony; seventh, Pilgrim John Alden, the young enthusiast.

Previous to sighting land Mistress Elizabeth Hopkins, wife of Master Stephen Hopkins, was delivered of a son, who, on account of the circumstances of his birth was named Oceanus, the first birth aboard the ship during the voyage. Later (November 27, 1620), Mistress White, sister to Dr. Fuller, gave birth to a son which is called Peregrine, the first child born in Cape Cod Harbor,[22] and the first-born English child in New England. There was another birth on the Mayflower December 22, 1620, while in Plymouth Harbor, son of Isaac Allerton, dead-born,[23] mother died February 25, 1621.

Scarcely had the Mayflower anchored in Cape Cod Harbor before sickness and death began their cruel work. Including the thirty-five days' stay in Cape Cod Harbor the voyagers had been one hundred and two days in coming from Plymouth, England, to Plymouth (New England), or one hundred and forty-five days from London. The condition of the Pilgrims did not improve after reaching Plymouth; their sickness and mortality can be best appreciated from Bradford's account; he says:[24] "But that which was most sadd & lamentable was, that in 2 or 3 moneths time halfe of their company dyed, espetialy in Jan: & February, being ye depth of winter, and wanting houses and other comforts; being infected with ye scurvie & other diseases, which this long vioyage & their inacomodate condition had brought upon them; so as ther dyed sometimes 2 or 3 of a day in ye foresaid time; that of 100 & odd persons scarce 50, remained. And of these in ye time of most distress, ther was but 6 or 7 sound persons who, to their great commendation be it spoken, spared no pains, night nor day, but with abundance of toyle and hazard of their own health, fetched them woode, made them fires, drest them meat, made their beads, washed their lothsome cloathes, cloathed & uncloathed them; in a word did all ye homly & necessarie offices for them wch deinty & quesie stomacks cannot endure to hear named."

Many guesses have been ventured as to the exact nature of this first illness. The overcrowding, the under-feeding, the trials, hardships and anxieties of the long voyage might be as favorable to the inception and development of one disease as another. There is every reason to believe that no infectious disease prevailed during the voyage. The only deaths were those of the seaman and William Butten, Doctor Fuller's assistant.

On November 11/21 a party of fifteen or sixteen men went ashore. On the 13/23 "many went ashore to refresh themselves, and the women to wash." An exploring party left on November 15/25, and was gone two days, during which time they followed Indians ten miles, found a store of buried corn and a big ship's kettle which they brought to ship. November 19/29 seamen went ashore. During all these trips it was necessary to wade in icy water up to the hips, and many are reported as having taken colds and coughs.

November 27/December 7, a party of twenty-four passengers, nine of the crew and the master of the ship, set out for land and a snow storm of six inches in depth forced them to remain on shore. They brought back corn, baskets, pottery, wickerware, etc., which they found buried in two graves and Indian houses.

December 4/14, the first death occurred, 17 days since the corn, kettle, etc., were brought on board. There were three deaths from illnesses as well as the death from drowning of Mistress Dorothy Bradford (December 7/17) during the thirty-five days the Mayflower lay in Cape Cod Harbor. The Mayflower reached Plymouth December 17/27, many reported sick, one of the Leyden party died December 21/31, another December 24/January 3. December 28/January 7, "Many ill from exposure." January 1/11, 1621, a death on Mayflower. January 8/18, another death. January 11/21, many ill aboard, Bradford and Carver ill on shore. On December 25, 1620 (January 4, 1621), the first house was started. It was about 20 feet square, and was a common rendezvous.

It was principally used for the sick, and may be well considered to be the first hospital erected in this country. From
this time the general sickness increased; there were 8 deaths
during January, 17 during February, 13 during March, and
6 for the rest of the year. That the sickness was brought
to the ship from shore would appear from Bradford's account, February 27/March 9: "The sickness and deaths of
the colonists on shore have steadily increased, and have ex-
tended to the ship, which has lost several of its petty officers,
including the master gunner, three quartermasters and cook,
and a third of the crew, many from scurvy." February 28/
March 10, he says: "The fifty-third day the ship has lain
in this harbor (Plymouth), and from the present rate of
sickness and death aboard, no present capacity or prospect
of getting away, those better being yet weak." March 24/
April 3, "Many still sick, more on the ship than on shore."
From this account it would appear that the sickness was of
an acute, highly contagious nature, that it did not manifest
itself until the passengers had gone ashore, drank the water,
and brought corn and utensils from the Indian camps; that
the sailors did not become ill until some of them had gone
on the exploration with the passengers. Assuming the disease to be other than acute tuberculosis, which has been
claimed to be the cause,[25] it must have been a disease whose
period of incubation was from ten to twenty days. Scurvy
we know existed, also acute coughs and colds, due to wetting
and exposure, but Dr. Fuller, Bradford, Winslow and others,
as well as the seamen, were well acquainted with the course
of scurvy and would not fear it. It is not contagious, and
there is little in the course of scurvy to suggest disgust in
nursing the same. An argument against tuberculosis
would appear from the fact that many recovered but were
quite weak for some time, i. e., a slow convalescence. It is
well established that the country about Massachusetts Bay
had been swept by an epidemic of a very infectious disease two years before the landing of the Pilgrims. What that
disease was can only be conjectured. Also in 1616 there had
been a pestilence among the Indians which was thought to
be either plague or smallpox, but which did not affect the

[267] English, although they lived and slept in the same cabins with the Indians.[26] Smallpox had been introduced into this country by the Spaniards in the early part of the sixteenth century.[27]

From the description gathered principally from Bradford's and Winslow's writings, as well as the history and course of the epidemic later at Salem, Charlestown and Dorchester, it would seem that the disease which caused the greatest mortality among the first settlers was either smallpox or typhus fever (plague), or a virulent form of typhoid. That there were cases of consumption, pneumonia, rheumatism and scurvy seems most natural under the circumstances. The most we know of the course of the sickness is that Bradford was reported very ill on January 11, 1621, and when he was elected as second Governor of Plymouth Colony in April, 1621, he was still too ill to take up the duties of the office. It is also known that the epidemic of sickness in 1634 was smallpox[28] and was fatal to many who had been exposed to the sickness in 1621. It is interesting to note that even at this early date consumption was considered a communicable disease. Frescatorius (1483-1553), who was the first to publish a description of typhus fever, says:[29] "Consumption is contagious, and is contracted by living with a phthisical person, by the gliding of the corrupted and putrefied juices (of the sick) into the lungs of the sound man." Measles and smallpox had been known from the middle of the ninth century.[30] From the knowledge which we possess of Dr. Fuller's education it is not unreasonable to assume that he was familiar with the writings and medical discoveries of the old writers. At London, and more especially at Leyden, he had every facility to consult their works. There is positive evidence that Doctor Fuller practiced bleeding, which was so universally employed at the beginning of the seventeenth century. Fuller did not limit his services to the settlers at New Plymouth. We find him dressing the wounds and curing the injuries of the Indians against whom Captain Standish proceeded in 1621. Also in 1622 upon the arrival of the Weston colonists, whom the Plymouth settlers had every reason to dislike, the sick and lame among them were

left at Plymouth by permission of the Governor, although
they had a surgeon in their party (Mr. Salisbury),[31] until
their health was restored by Doctor Fuller, which he did
without pay.[32] The wife and daughter of Samuel Fuller were
passengers on the Anne in 1623. Two children were born
in this country, Mercy, and Samuel who in 1694 was the
first minister in Plymouth church. He had seven children,
one of whom, Isaac, was the first physician in Middleboro.
There is little to relate in the history of the Colony during
the years 1623-1627. More or less sickness prevailed, yet
there was no special epidemic. One event is recorded which
shows that Doctor Fuller possessed a heart which was most
tender and charitable towards his fellowmen. A certain. Mr.
Lyford came to the Colony in 1624 in the guise of a minister,
but who in reality was a hypocrite and traitor. His schem-
ing was frustrated and he was confronted with the evidence
of his duplicity. At first he denied the charges, but later
publicly confessed his sins in the church, and so great and
sincere was the appearance of his repentance "that Samuel
Fuller and some other tender-hearted men were so taken with
his signs of sorrow and repentance, as they professed they
would fall upon their knees to have his censure released."[33]
Fuller's charity was misplaced, for Lyford's reformation did
not last two months. In the affairs of trade and government
of the Colonists, Doctor Fuller, although one of Governor
Bradford's councillors, appears to have taken little part. He
gave bonds with others, to the company of adventurers in
England, yet he does not seem to be held by rigid demands
of that bond. His mission and sacrifice were greater than
that of worldly gain and his chief recompense was the love
and gratitude of those who sought his sympathy and advice
in their great trials, both physical and spiritual. When
Bradford became Governor, Doctor Fuller was one of his
selected councillors together with four others.

Doctor Fuller, unlike many of the early settlers, did not
combine disputation nor bigotry with his religious views.
To him a sick person was a call to duty, whether it came
from Puritan or Pilgrim, Huguenot or Catholic, friend or
foe, white man or Indian, all alike received the fullest meas-

[267] ure of which he was capable. We are not surprised, therefore, to find him laboring among the Puritans of the settlements at Salem, also at Dorchester and Charlestown in 1628,
'29 and '30. When Governor Endicott arrived in Salem there
was much sickness of an infectious nature among the pas-
[268] sengers. This sickness spread to those on land and many
died, " Some of ye scurvie, other of an infectious feavure,
which continued some time amongst them (though our people
(the Plymouth settlement) escaped it." Endicott wrote to
Governor Bradford begging the services of Doctor Fuller
whom he had heard had " cured diverse of ye scurvie, and
others of other diseases by letting blood, & other means."
In view of the strained relationship which existed between
the Pilgrims and Puritans up to this time Doctor Fuller's
visit had an important bearing upon the affairs of the whole
Colony. Governor Endicott wrote Governor Bradford, " I ac-
knowledge myself much bound to you for your kind love and
care in sending Mr. Fuller among us, and rejoice much that
I am by him satisfied touching your judgments of the out-
ward form of God's worship. It is as far as I can gather,
no other than is warranted by the evidence of truth, and the
same which I have professed and maintained ever since the
Lord in mercy revealed Himself unto me, being far from the
common report that has been spread of you touching that
particular." [34]

From this letter it is evident that Doctor Fuller improved
his opportunities and fully converted Governor Endicott from
the prejudices and jealousies which he held concerning the
Plymouth Settlement. It is worthy of note that Mrs. Endicott died during one of these visits of Doctor Fuller. Governor Winthrop's settlers shared the fate of all the other expeditions to the Colonies, and so great was the sickness among
them at Charlestown that Doctor Fuller was requested to aid
them in their distress, which he promptly did, rendering good
assistance and earning the thanks of Governor Winthrop and
his Colony.

In June, 1630, Doctor Fuller wrote: [35] " I have been to
Matapan (now Dorchester) and let some twenty of those people blood." Again, in August, 1630, while at Charlestown he

writes: [36] "There is come hither a ship (with cattle and more passengers) on Saturday last which brings this news out of England; that the plague is sore, both in the city and country, also there is like to be a good dearth in the land by reason of the dry season—the sad news here is that many are sick and many are dead—I here but lose time and long to be at home. I can do them no good, for I want drugs and things fitting to work with." In these letters we find positive proof that Doctor Fuller knew that the infectious nature of the disease called for other remedies than bleeding. Much surprise and confusion has been manifested by many writers over the fact that Doctor Fuller bled the sick people of that period, yet bleeding was a well authorized treatment for typhus fever during the seventeenth century,[37] a fact which strongly suggests the sickness prevailing.

Governor Endicott in his memoirs [38] says: " Such was the great mortality among them (Endicott's party) during this first winter after their arrival arising from the rigors of untried climate, and their being badly fit and badly lodged that there were scarcely found in the settlement well persons enough to nurse and console the sick—to enhance their distress they were destitute of any regular medical assistance." Doctor Fuller was a man of keen observation and good reasoning. In writing to Governor Bradford while he was yet among the people at Dorchester (1630) he says: " I have had conferences with them all till I was weary. The Governor (Endicott) is a goodly wise and humble gentleman and very discreet, and of a firm and good temper. We have some privy enemies in the bay but (blessed be God) more friends,—the Governor had conference with me, both in private and before sundrie others—the Governor told me he hoped we will not be wanting in helping them, so that I think you will be sent for." [39] The great influence which these visits of Doctor Fuller to the Endicott Settlement had upon the affairs of the early progress of this country has never been fully set forth. There had been much disappointment in England over the result of the enterprise sent out here. Those who had backed the venture financially had received little or no return. The meagre exports from this country had been seized. Enemies had circulated many discouraging rumors in England concerning the objects and doings of the planters in New England. Winslow, Allerton and Standish had made repeated trips to England for support, but with little success. The Indians were being incited to hostilities, and finally the arrival of the Endicott party who brought with them prejudices and unfriendliness towards the Plymouth settlers. After Fuller had gone among them on his visit of mercy and help, all this changed. Endicott sent back to England a report setting forth in most favorable terms the state of affairs here, as well as a glowing account of the climate, the country and its resources. The result was a changed sentiment in England, an increased confidence in the Plymouth settlers and the active co-operation at home of men of wealth and position with a greater disposition towards emigration to this country, and consequently a rapid, vigorous growth of many new colonies which meant the complete success and permanency of the settlement in the new world. His successors in the healing art, if none others, might well provide a suitable memorial of this good physician's visits of mercy to the pestilent-stricken settlers of infant Salem, Dorchester and Boston.

In the epidemic of smallpox which prevailed in 1633 many fell very sick, and about twenty died, men, women and children, including many of the old settlers from Holland, among whom was Samuel Fuller (after he had much helped others) and "had been a great help and comforte unto them; as in his faculties, so otherwise, being a deacon in ye church, a man godly, and forward to doe good, being much missed after his death; and he and ye rest of their brethren much lemented by them, and caused much sadness & mourning amongst them." [40] This disease was also very fatal among the Indians from all the adjoining places. A curious fact in relation to this epidemic was that it had been prophesied by the Indians in May on account of the great quantities of a sort of fly, about the size of wasps or bumble bees, which came out of holes in the ground, and filled the woods, eating the green things and making a constant yelling noise, deafening to hear. These insects (locusts?) were unknown to the English. The epidemic followed in June, July and August during the heat of summer. Notwithstanding the many trials, hardships and toils to which a physician is subjected even in these days of conveniences and luxuries, it is both gratifying and significant to find this early physician acting as the guardian of the future welfare of the community by perpetuating learning among its children. In his will he mentions four youths entrusted to his care who were to be returned to their parents at Charlestown and Dorchester. This will, both on account of the fact that it is the first will probated in this country as well as the many points mentioned therein touching the life, work and character of Doctor Fuller is here abstracted as follows: "

" I Samuel Fuller the Elder being sick & weake, but by the mercie of God in pfect memory ordaine this my last will and testmt. I doe bequeath the Education of my children to my Brother Will Wright & his wife, onely that my daughter Mercy be & remaine to good-wife Wallen so long as she will keepe her at a reasonable charge. But if it shall please God to recover my wife out of her weake state of sickness then my children to be with her or disposed by her. I desire my Brother Wright may have the bringing up of a childe comitted to my charge, called Sarah Converse, but if he refuse then I comend her to my loving neighbor and brother in Christ Thomas Prince.

" Item. Whereas Eliz. Cowles was submitted to my educacion by her father and mother still living at Charlestowne, my will is that she conveniently appelled & returne to her ffather or mother. And for George ffoster being placed wth me by his parents still living at Sagos, my will is that he be restored to his mother. Item. I give to my son Samuel my house and land at the Smelt river; I order certain portions of my estate (naming them) to be sold to educate my two children Samuel & Mercy. I give land adjoining Mr. Isaac Allerton's to my son Samuel and also land on Strawbury hill given to me by Edward Bircher, if Mr. Roger Williams refuse to accept it as he has formerly done. Item. My will is that my cozen Samuel, goe away with his stock of cattle and swine without any further recconing. Item. My Estates, and cattle with my two servants Thomas Symons & Rob't Cowles be

[269] employed for the good of my two children, by my Brother Wright and Priscilla his wife. I give to the church of God at Plymouth the first cow calfe that my brown cow shall have. I give to my sister Alice Bradford twelve shillings to buy her a pair of gloves. Whatever is due to me from Capt. Standish I give unto his children. Item. That a paire of gloves of 5sh be bestowed on Mr. Jno. Winthrop Gov. of the Massachusetts. Item. Whereas Capt. John Endicott oweth me two pounds of Beaver, I give it to his sonne. It. My will is that my children be ruled by my overseers in marriage. It. I give unto John, Jenny & Joh. Winslow each of them a pair of gloves of five shillings. It. I give unto Mr. Heeke, the full sum of twenty shillings. I give unto Mr. William Brewster my best hat and band wch I never wore. I give to Rebecca Prince 2 sch 6d to buy her a pair of gloves. My will is that in case my son Samuel die before he come into inheritance of my estate then they are to go to my kinsman Samuel Fuller now in the house with me. I appoint my son Samuel my executor, and Mr. Edward Winslow, Mr. William Bradford & Mr. Thomas Prince my overseers. To my daughter Mercy one Bible with a black cover. It. Whatsoever Mr. Roger Williams is indebted to me upon my booke for physick I fuly give him."

"Memoranda—Whereas the widow Ring submitted to me the oversight of her sonne Andrew my will is that Mr. Price take charge of him."

Fac-Simile Autograph.
Very rare.

The widow of Samuel Fuller and her son Samuel joined in a gift (1644) to the church of Plymouth for the use of a minister the land (half an acre) once owned and occupied by Doctor Fuller, and upon which the parsonage house of Harvey W. Weston now stands.⁴ Mrs. Fuller is mentioned as one of the earliest women practitioners of midwifery in this country. The town records of Rehoboth, Massachusetts, July 3, 1663, says, "Voted, and agreed that—Mrs. Bridget Fuller of Plymouth should be sent to, to see if she be willing to come and dwell among us to attend on the office of midwife, to answer the town's necessity, which at present is great."

This invitation was not accepted, as she died at Plymouth [269] the next year.[43] Her son Samuel was offered the call to the church at Rehoboth at the same time. The son Samuel became a clergyman and was the first minister of the church at Middleboro, Massachusetts. He married a granddaughter of Elder Brewster.[44] His daughter Mercy married Ralp James.

On the death of Doctor Fuller an early writer[45] says: " In his medical character, and for his christian virtues and unfeigned piety Dr. Fuller was held in the highest estimation, and was resorted to as a father and wise counselor during the perils of his day. He was finally one of the several heads of families who died of a fever which prevailed in Plymouth in the summer of 1633, and was most deeply lamented by all the colonists."

Doctor Fuller's library contained only twenty-seven books, among which are mentioned two dictionaries and " Peter Martyr on Rome." It is safe to suppose that the well-stocked libraries of Brewster, Winslow and Bradford were freely open to the use of Doctor Fuller. Although medical literature must have been very scarce in those days, the physical endurance required for a day's labor was hardly calculated to encourage much leisure reading. Meagre as were the literary advantages of the early colonists, one of the most prominent characteristics of the people was the solicitude for the education of the children. New England's First Fruits published in London in 1643 says: " One of the next things we longed for, and looked after, was to advance learning and perpetuate it to Posterity."[46] It is to this spirit that the founding of Harvard College at such an early period (1638) can be ascribed, a movement in which Samuel Fuller must have been an early and important factor. In this connection it may be said that the influence which Doctor Fuller had exercised for the cause of education was continued by his good wife, and the first court record which alludes to schools in this country [270] says that it was ordered by the court in 1635 " that Benjamine Eaton (a lad 8 years old) with his mother's consent, is put to Bridget Fuller, being to keep him at school for two years, and employ him after in such service as she saw fit, and he

[270] shall be fit for." [47] Modernity is apt to lay claim to all that is good and noble in the many walks of life, forgetful of the many hardships, sacrifices and trials which have been endured and overcome in its completion. Let us hope that the one profession above all others whose whole life is one of self-sacrifice and charity will not be unmindful of the good work of its pioneers.

History affords fewer examples more worthy of honoring or more creditably representing the self-sacrificing, broad-minded, truly charitable Christian physician than the life practiced by Doctor Samuel Fuller among the first settlers in this country. How fittingly apply the words of the Master, " Greater love hath no man than this, that a man lay down his life for his friends."

REFERENCES.

1. Baas' History of Medicine. Translation.

2. New England Historical and Genealogical Register, vol. 35.

3. Aubrey, History of England, vol. 2.

4. The Mayflower and Her Log. Ames.

5. Mail and Express, New York, 1896.

6. Davis' Genealogical Register of Plymouth Families.

7. Rev. Edward Everett Hale, New England Magazine, September, 1889.

8. Davis' Ancient Landmarks of Plymouth.

9. Ibid.

10. American Medical Biography, by James Thacher, M. D.

11. The Transit of Civilization, by Edward Eggleston.

12. Boston Medical and Surgical Journal, vol. CXLVII, No. 21.

13. The Bradford History of Plymouth Plantation.

14. The Mayflower and Her Log. Ames.

15. American Medical Biography, by James Thacher, M. D., 1828.

16. Ibid.

17. Ibid.

18. The Mayflower and Her Log. Ames.

19. The Bradford History of the Plymouth Plantation. [270]

20. New England Magazine, February, 1897, by Edward E. Cornwall, M. D.

21. Bradford in Mourt's Relation.

22. The Mayflower and Her Log.

23. Ibid.

24. The Bradford History, from Original Manuscript.

25. Dr. Edward E. Cornwall, New England Magazine, February, 1897.

26. History and Antiquities of Boston, by Samuel G. Drake, A. M.

27. Osler, Practice of Medicine.

28. Morton: New Engand's Memorial.

29. De Morbis Contagiosis, lib. II, cap. IX, Dr. Mead.

30. The Origin and Growth of the Healing Art.

31. The Pilgrim Republic, by Goodwin.

32. Youngs' Chronicles of the Pilgrim Fathers.

33. The Bradford History of the Plymouth Plantation.

34. John Brown, Pilgrim Fathers in New England.

35. Massachusetts Historical Collection III.

36. Massachusetts Historical Collection III.

37. Peppers' System of Medicine.

38. New England Historical and Genealogical Register, vol. I.

39. Massachusetts Historical Collection III.

40. The Bradford History of Plymouth Plantation.

41. New England Historical and Genealogical Register, vol. IV.

42. Davis' Ancient Landmarks of Plymouth.

43. History of Medicine in the United States, by Francis Randolph Packard, M. D.

44. Genealogical Dictionary of New England Families, by Savage, vol. II.

45. American Medical Biography, by James Thacher, M. D.

46. Harvard Graduate Magazine, vol. III, No. 9, Henry Cabot Lodge.

47. Davis' Genealogical Register of Plymouth Families.